The Marriage Cancer

Recognizing and handling emotional abuse in marriage

By

Inspira

Table of Contents

Introduction

"Emotional abuse is the silent killer of love, slowly suffocating the spirit and leaving scars that may never heal. It is a weapon that is wielded with words and actions, undermining the very foundation of trust and intimacy in a marriage. The bruises may not be visible, but the pain is real. Victims are left trapped in a cycle of despair and self-doubt." - Unknown

Amidst the grand tapestry of human relationships, marriage is often hailed as a sacred bond. A sanctuary where two souls unite in love, commitment, and mutual support. It is a journey filled with hope and dreams, a partnership that promises to weather life's storms together. However, behind closed doors, some marriages bear witness to a darker reality. One that shatters these ideals and erodes the very essence of love. This book shines a light on the profound issue of emotional abuse within the institution of marriage. It offers understanding, guidance, and healing for those who have endured its torment.

Consider the story of Sarah. At first glance, Sarah appeared to have it all—a successful career, a loving husband, and a beautiful home. Yet, beneath the facade of perfection, a different reality loomed. Her husband, Daniel, was an expert manipulator, adept at exploiting her vulnerabilities to gain control over every aspect of their relationship. Through a relentless barrage of belittling comments, gaslighting, and emotional manipulation, Daniel wielded his power over Sarah. This resulted in dismantling her self-worth and independence. Day by day, she found herself walking on eggshells, tiptoeing through an emotional minefield, desperately seeking to appease her tormentor.

Sarah's story is just one among countless tales of emotional abuse that unfold behind closed doors every day. Emotional abuse, unlike physical abuse, leaves no visible marks, making it all the more insidious. It seeps into the very fabric of a relationship, poisoning the wellspring of love and affection. Victims are left questioning their own sanity, struggling to reconcile the stark contrast between the person they once were and the hollow shell they have become.

This book includes the stories of various victims of emotional abuse, but their names have been changed to maintain their confidentiality. The book is a testament to the courage and resilience of those who have endured emotional abuse, offering hope and understanding to those who find themselves trapped in the suffocating grip of an abusive marriage. By shedding light on the various forms of emotional abuse and their profound impact on individuals and relationships, it aims to empower victims to recognize the signs, break free from the cycle of abuse, and rebuild their lives.

This book is not solely focused on the victims. It also extends a compassionate hand to those who perpetrate emotional abuse, encouraging them to confront their own behaviors, seek help, and embark on a journey of personal transformation. By fostering understanding and empathy, this book aims to break the cycle of abuse, offering a glimmer of hope for couples willing to embark on the difficult path toward healing and reconciliation.

In the pages that follow, I invite you to explore the complex world of emotional abuse within the context of marriage. We acknowledge the pain and turmoil that emotional abuse inflicts. However, we also emphasize the power of resilience, self-discovery, and healing. Let this book serve as a guiding light, offering solace, validation, and practical advice for those who have endured emotional abuse.

Chapter 1: What, how and why?

Sub-chapter 1: Understanding emotional abuse

Jane's heart pounded in her chest as she stood in front of the mirror, meticulously applying concealer to hide the bruise on her cheek. Her husband's cutting words still echoed in her mind, as fresh tears welled up in her eyes. She couldn't understand how the person she once loved had become her worst enemy, inflicting wounds that cut deeper than any physical pain. Jane was trapped in the web of emotional abuse, a silent torment that left her questioning her worth and her very sanity.

Jane's story is an example of emotional abuse, which is a form of psychological manipulation and control that leaves no visible scars but wreaks havoc on the emotional well-being of its victims. It takes various insidious forms, such as verbal attacks, humiliation, constant criticism, gaslighting, and isolation. Unlike physical abuse, emotional abuse chips away at a person's self-esteem, distorting their perception of reality and leaving them feeling powerless and trapped within their own minds.

Within the confines of marriage, emotional abuse often thrives behind closed doors, hidden from the prying eyes of the outside world. The abuser, driven by a need for power and control, exploits the intimate nature of the relationship to manipulate and dominate their partner. It can manifest in ways such as constant belittlement, control over finances, monitoring communication, withholding affection or intimacy, and fostering a climate of fear and intimidation. The victim, bound by love, societal expectations, and the hope of change, may endure years of emotional torment before finding the strength to break free.

Jennifer was a woman who once radiated confidence and joy, found herself trapped in a marriage that suffocated her spirit. Her husband's constant criticism of her appearance, belittlement of her achievements, and refusal to acknowledge her worth left her feeling like a shadow of her former self. Jennifer's story serves as a stark reminder that emotional abuse erodes the very core of one's identity, leaving them feeling unworthy and unlovable.

We are also compelled to give the story of Robert. He was a man who believed in the strength of his love and the power of forgiveness, but struggled in silence as his wife systematically isolated him from his family and friends. Her constant need for control and manipulation left him feeling isolated and disconnected, eroding the once vibrant bond they shared. Robert's story highlights that emotional abuse knows no gender boundaries and can affect anyone, regardless of societal expectations or stereotypes.

Unknown to most of us, emotional abuse within marriage is a silent epidemic that inflicts profound pain and suffering on its victims. For instance, in the United States, a report published by the National Intimate Partner & Sexual Violence Survey (NISVS) in 2011 found that 50% of Americans had undergone emotional abuse from their partners during their lifetime [1].

By understanding the nature of emotional abuse, recognizing its manifestations within intimate relationships, and exploring the underlying causes, we can begin to break the cycle and offer support to those affected.

Subchapter 2: Watch out!

Through various life experiences, we can attest to the fact that emotional abuse within a marriage can be crippling, leaving lasting scars on the emotional and mental well-being of the victim. Using stories of people that have given us permission to share them, we will show you that emotional abuse is a monster that we all need to address.

Emotional abuse chips away at a person's sense of self-worth, leaving them with deep-seated feelings of inadequacy, shame, and self-doubt. Rachel, a survivor of emotional abuse, recalls how her husband's constant criticism shattered her self-esteem, causing her to question her own abilities and lose confidence in her decision-making.

Victims of emotional abuse are often isolated from their support networks, leaving them feeling alone and trapped in their suffering. Luke, who endured years of emotional abuse, recounts how his wife systematically distanced him from his friends and family, leaving him with a sense of profound loneliness and a lack of emotional support.

The constant barrage of verbal attacks, threats, and manipulation creates an environment of fear and uncertainty, leading many victims to develop anxiety disorders and depression. Laura vividly recalls the anxiety attacks she experienced whenever her husband unleashed his anger, causing her to live in a perpetual state of fear and apprehension.

The effects of emotional abuse extend far beyond the immediate pain and trauma, often leaving lasting imprints on the lives of those who have endured it. Let's now examine some of the long-term effects that emotional abuse can have on marriages.

Emotional abuse erodes the foundations of trust, intimacy, and emotional connection within a marriage. The repeated betrayal and manipulation create a deep-seated mistrust that is difficult to repair. Jacinda, whose husband used gaslighting tactics, struggled to trust her own perceptions, leading to a breakdown in the emotional bond they once shared.

Victims can also go into self-imposed isolation as a means of self-protection. Many victims withdraw from social interactions, becoming emotionally guarded and hesitant to form new relationships. This reminds me of James. After leaving an emotionally abusive marriage, James found it challenging to trust and open up to new partners, fearing a repetition of the pain he had experienced.

Unknown to many people, emotional abuse within a marriage also has far-reaching consequences for children and the broader family unit. Research shows that in families where a woman is abused, there is a 60-75% likelihood of abuse on the children [2]. Witnessing their parents' toxic relationship can also leave lasting emotional scars on children, affecting their self-esteem, ability to form healthy relationships, and overall well-being. Emma, a young woman who grew up in an emotionally abusive household, struggled with her own sense of self-worth and experienced difficulties in establishing healthy boundaries in her adult relationships.

These personal stories serve as poignant reminders of the profound and long-lasting effects emotional abuse can have on marriages. The pain and devastation caused by emotional abuse cannot be overstated, and it is crucial to acknowledge and address these effects in order to facilitate healing and promote healthier relationship dynamics.

Conclusion

Jane's harrowing experience and the stories of Rachel, Luke, Laura, Jacinda, James, and Emma shed light on the devastating impact of emotional abuse within marriages. Emotional abuse, although invisible, leaves profound scars on the victims, eroding their self-esteem, isolating them from support networks, and instilling fear and anxiety. It undermines trust, intimacy, and emotional connection, leading to long-lasting damage in relationships. The consequences extend beyond the couple to affect children and the broader family unit, perpetuating a cycle of pain and dysfunction.

In the next chapter, we will delve into the mind of an emotionally abusive person, exploring their thoughts, conceptions, misconceptions, and mental frameworks.

Understanding the dynamics from the perspective of the abuser can offer insights into the underlying causes and help develop strategies for intervention and prevention. By gaining this understanding, we can work towards creating a society where emotional abuse is recognized, condemned, and eradicated, fostering healthier relationships built on respect, trust, and empathy.

Chapter Summary

- Emotional abuse in marriage is a form of psychological manipulation and control that leaves no visible scars but wreaks havoc on the emotional well-being of its victims.

- Abusers exploit the intimate nature of the relationship to manipulate and dominate their partner, leading to constant belittlement, control over finances, isolation, and fostering fear and intimidation.

- Victims often struggle with feelings of unworthiness and unlovability, and endure years of emotional torment before finding the strength to break free.

- Emotional abuse knows no gender boundaries and can affect anyone.

- The long-term effects of emotional abuse include the deterioration of trust, intimacy, and emotional connection within the marriage.

Chapter 2: Mind vs matter

The phenomenon of emotional abuse within marriages is a deeply complex issue that requires a comprehensive understanding of the motivations, mental frameworks, and mindsets of individuals who perpetrate emotional abuse. In this chapter, we will delve into the intricate workings of the emotionally abusive mind, exploring various psychological theories and the role of childhood trauma, upbringing, and schooling in shaping the behavior of emotional abusers.

Sub-chapter 1: Psychological Theories and Motivations of Emotional Abuse

The Power and Control Model is a psychological theory that provides valuable insights into the motivations behind emotional abuse [3]. According to this model, emotional abusers seek power and control over their partners as a means of compensating for their own feelings of inadequacy or insecurity [3]. By exerting control through manipulation and emotional abuse, they attempt to maintain a sense of power and superiority.

Attachment theory offers another lens through which to understand the dynamics of emotional abuse [4]. Individuals with insecure attachment styles, characterized by a fear of abandonment or rejection, may resort to emotional abuse as a means of maintaining control and avoiding the perceived threat of rejection [4]. These individuals often struggle with deep-seated fears of intimacy and vulnerability, which contribute to their abusive behavior.

Cognitive distortions and dysfunctional beliefs play a significant role in the mental frameworks of emotional abusers. These individuals may hold distorted views about relationships, such as beliefs that their own needs are paramount, a sense of entitlement, and a lack of empathy for their partners. Cognitive distortions, such as minimizing or justifying their abusive behavior, allow emotional abusers to rationalize their actions and avoid taking responsibility for the harm they cause.

Sub-chapter 2: Mental Processes of Emotional Abusers

Emotional abusers frequently employ manipulation tactics and gaslighting techniques to exert control over their victims. Gaslighting involves distorting or denying the victim's perception of reality, making them doubt their own experiences and sanity. By manipulating their partner's thoughts, emotions, and perceptions, emotional abusers ensure compliance and exert dominance.

Projection and blame-shifting are common behaviors among emotional abusers. They often project their own insecurities, flaws, and negative emotions onto their partners, deflecting responsibility for their actions. By shifting blame, emotional abusers make their partners feel responsible for their abusive behavior or emotional distress, thus avoiding accountability and maintaining a sense of superiority.

Emotional abusers often employ intermittent reinforcement as a manipulation tactic. They alternate between periods of love, affection, and kindness, and periods of emotional abuse. This creates a cycle of hope and despair for the victim, leaving them constantly striving for the abuser's validation and affection. The intermittent reinforcement of positive behavior makes it challenging for the victim to break free from the abusive relationship.

Sub-chapter 3: The Impact of Childhood Trauma, Upbringing, and Schooling

Childhood trauma, such as experiencing physical or emotional abuse, neglect, or witnessing domestic violence, can significantly contribute to the development of emotional abusers. These early experiences can distort their understanding of healthy relationships and perpetuate a cycle of abuse. Emotional abusers who have experienced trauma may replicate the abusive patterns they witnessed or endured as a means of coping or gaining a sense of control.

The upbringing and family dynamics of emotional abusers can also shape their behavior. Growing up in an environment where emotional abuse is normalized or witnessed can perpetuate the cycle of abuse across generations. Children who observe emotional abuse between their parents may internalize these behaviors as acceptable or normal, leading them to become emotional abusers themselves in their adult relationships.

While childhood experiences play a significant role, societal factors, including schooling, can also contribute to the development of emotional abusers. Toxic masculinity norms, rigid gender roles, and a lack of education on healthy relationships can perpetuate abusive behaviors. In some cases, individuals may learn manipulative tactics or abusive patterns from peers or media, further reinforcing their abusive mindset.

Conclusion

As we conclude this chapter, we will remind you that understanding the motivations, mental frameworks, and mindsets of emotional abusers is crucial in addressing and preventing emotional abuse. Psychological theories shed light on the power dynamics, attachment styles, and cognitive distortions that contribute to emotional abuse. Additionally, childhood trauma, upbringing, and societal factors play significant roles in shaping the behavior of emotional abusers. By gaining insights into the mental processes of emotional abusers, we can develop strategies to challenge and change abusive behaviors. Interventions focused on increasing self-awareness, empathy, and healthy coping mechanisms can help individuals break free from the patterns of emotional abuse and develop healthier relationship dynamics. Education, awareness, and fostering a culture of respect and equality are key in preventing emotional abuse and creating safe and nurturing relationships.

Chapter Summary

•   Emotional abuse within marriages is a complex issue requiring an understanding of the motivations, mental frameworks, and mindsets of abusers.

•   Psychological theories, such as the Power and Control Model, Attachment Theory, and Cognitive Distortions, provide insights into the motivations behind emotional abuse.

- Emotional abusers employ manipulation tactics, gaslighting, projection, blame-shifting, and intermittent reinforcement to exert control and maintain power over their victims.

- Childhood trauma, upbringing, and societal factors, including schooling, can shape the behavior of emotional abusers, perpetuating a cycle of abuse. Understanding these factors is crucial in developing strategies to address and prevent emotional abuse.

Chapter 3: Am I a statistic?

Have you ever found yourself questioning the dynamics of your relationships? Do you sometimes feel overwhelmed, drained, or constantly on edge in the presence of certain individuals? If so, you may be experiencing emotional abuse, a subtle yet destructive form of mistreatment that can leave lasting scars on one's emotional well-being. In this chapter, we will delve into the intricacies of emotional abuse, exploring the tests, signs, and an emotional abuse checklist that can help you recognize this harmful behavior.

Imagine this: Sophia, a successful professional, had always been confident and assertive. However, ever since she started dating Daniel, her self-esteem has gradually diminished. Daniel constantly criticizes her appearance, dismisses her achievements, and isolates her from her friends and family. Sophia's once vibrant personality has been replaced by anxiety and self-doubt. In this chapter, we will unravel the emotional abuse hidden within Sophia's relationship, shedding light on the methods that perpetrators employ to exert control and manipulate their victims.

In this chapter, we will embark on a journey to understand

emotional abuse in its various forms. We will begin by discussing the tests for emotional abuse, which can help individuals evaluate their relationships and identify potential abuse. Understanding these tests is crucial, as emotional abuse often manifests subtly, making it difficult to recognize and address.

Next, we will explore five common signs of emotional abuse. By recognizing these signs, individuals can gain insight into their experiences and validate their concerns. Moreover, identifying these signs can serve as a wake-up call, empowering victims to take steps toward healing and reclaiming their autonomy.

Finally, we will provide an emotional abuse checklist—a comprehensive tool that can assist individuals in assessing the health of their relationships. This checklist will outline specific behaviors and patterns commonly associated with emotional abuse. By systematically evaluating these elements, readers can gain a clearer perspective on their own experiences and make informed decisions about their relationships.

Subchapter 1: Tests for Emotional Abuse

Emotional abuse is often insidious, gradually eroding one's self-esteem and emotional well-being. To help individuals determine if they are in an emotionally abusive relationship, several tests have been developed. We will explore some of these tests, including the Emotional Abuse Test and the Power and Control Wheel, and discuss how they can be utilized to evaluate one's relationship dynamics.

The Emotional Abuse Test: The Emotional Abuse Test is designed to help individuals evaluate their experiences within a relationship and assess whether emotional abuse is present [5]. This test typically consists of a series of questions that explore various aspects of the relationship, such as communication patterns, respect, control, and emotional well-being. By answering these questions honestly, individuals can gain insight into the dynamics of their relationship and recognize potential signs of emotional abuse. The Emotional Abuse Test assesses behaviors that are often associated with emotional abuse, such as constant criticism, humiliation, manipulation, control, isolation, and gaslighting. It prompts individuals to reflect on their partner's actions and their own emotional state within the relationship. The test serves as a guide to help individuals identify patterns of mistreatment that may be negatively impacting their well-being. You can find the quiz on this link.

Power and Control Wheel: The Power and Control Wheel is a visual representation of the various tactics and behaviors employed by individuals who exert power and control over their partners in an abusive relationship [6]. It was originally developed to illustrate the dynamics of domestic violence but can also be applied to emotional abuse. The Power and Control Wheel consists of a circular diagram with different sections, each representing a specific form of control or abuse as shown in figure 2. These sections often include physical violence, intimidation, isolation, minimizing, denying, blaming, using children, economic abuse, and emotional abuse. Emotional abuse is a significant component of the wheel and encompasses behaviors such as degradation, threats, manipulation, and control.

Figure 2: The Power and Control Wheel adapted from Charvis and Hill (2009) [6]

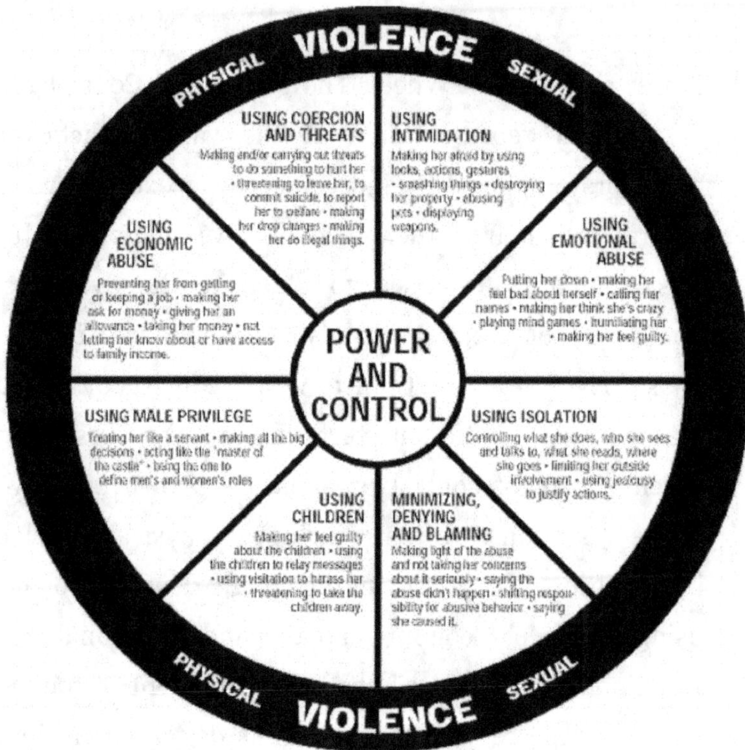

Both the Emotional Abuse Test and the Power and Control Wheel provide individuals with a structured approach to evaluate their relationship dynamics. They encourage self-reflection and help individuals identify potential signs of emotional abuse that may be affecting their well-being. These tests are valuable resources that raise awareness and prompt individuals to take action in seeking support, setting boundaries, and potentially leaving an abusive relationship. It is important to note that professional assistance from counselors or support services should be sought if emotional abuse is suspected.

Subchapter 2: Five Signs of Emotional Abuse

Recognizing the signs of emotional abuse is a crucial step toward breaking free from its destructive grip. In this section, we will delve into five key signs that may indicate emotional abuse: constant criticism and belittlement, manipulation and control, isolation from support systems, gaslighting, and emotional blackmail [7]. By understanding these signs, individuals can gain clarity and begin the healing process.

One of the most prevalent signs of emotional abuse is constant criticism and belittlement. In an emotionally abusive marriage, the spouse may consistently find fault in their partner's actions, appearance, or choices, often using derogatory language or insults [7]. This behavior undermines the victim's self-esteem and self-worth, leading them to feel inadequate, worthless, and constantly on edge. The abuser may employ subtle put-downs or outright attacks, making the victim doubt their abilities and question their own value.

Emotional abusers often exert control over their spouse

through manipulation tactics. They may employ various strategies to ensure compliance and dominance within the relationship. This manipulation can manifest as emotional blackmail, where the abuser uses threats, emotional manipulation, or coercion to manipulate the victim's actions or decisions. They may manipulate the victim's emotions, making them feel guilty or responsible for the abuser's behavior or emotional state. By controlling the victim's thoughts, feelings, and actions, the abuser establishes a power dynamic that leaves the victim feeling trapped and powerless.

Isolation from support systems is a common tactic employed by emotional abusers to maintain control over their spouse. They may strategically isolate the victim from family, friends, or other sources of support, creating a dependency on the abuser for emotional connection and validation [7]. The abuser may discourage or prevent the victim from maintaining outside relationships, instilling feelings of loneliness and helplessness. By cutting off the victim's support networks, the abuser gains greater control and makes it more challenging for the victim to seek assistance or escape the abusive environment.

Gaslighting is a manipulative technique used by emotional abusers to make their victims doubt their own reality. The abuser may deny or minimize their hurtful behavior, invalidate the victim's emotions, or distort facts and events. Gaslighting can leave the victim feeling confused, disoriented, and uncertain of their own perceptions. By manipulating the victim's sense of reality, the abuser maintains control and power over the relationship. This insidious tactic undermines the victim's confidence and fosters a sense of self-doubt, making it difficult for them to recognize and address the abuse.

Emotional blackmail is another destructive sign of emotional abuse. It involves the abuser using threats, manipulation, or emotional pressure to control their spouse's actions or decisions. They may employ tactics such as threatening to leave the relationship, harm themselves, or withhold love and affection unless the victim complies with their demands. This form of manipulation instills fear, guilt, and a sense of obligation in the victim, leaving them trapped in a cycle of compliance to avoid negative consequences [7]. Emotional blackmail creates a toxic environment where the victim's needs and desires are disregarded, and their autonomy is undermined.

These five signs of emotional abuse highlight the destructive nature of this form of mistreatment within a marriage. Recognizing these signs is crucial for victims to break free from the cycle of abuse and seek the support they need to regain their emotional well-being and independence. If you resonate with these signs or suspect you may be experiencing emotional abuse, reaching out to a professional counselor, support group, or helpline can provide guidance and assistance in navigating your situation and working towards a healthier future.

Subchapter 3: Emotional Abuse Checklist

To facilitate self-reflection and assessment, an emotional abuse checklist can be an invaluable resource. This section will present a comprehensive checklist that encompasses various dimensions of emotional abuse, such as verbal aggression, social isolation, financial control, and psychological manipulation. By evaluating their relationships using this checklist, readers can obtain a comprehensive picture of their experiences and make informed decisions about their emotional well-being.

Using this checklist can help married individuals assess their relationships and identify potential signs of emotional abuse. Please note that this checklist is not an official diagnostic tool but rather a resource to raise awareness and prompt reflection. Consider each item carefully and honestly evaluate your experiences within your marriage.

Figure 3: The emotional abuse checklist

Item	Explanation	Yes	No
Constant criticism and belittlement	Does your spouse frequently criticize or demean you? Do they consistently belittle your thoughts, feelings, or accomplishments, leaving you feeling inadequate or worthless?		
Manipulation and control	Does your spouse manipulate your emotions or exert control over your actions? Are you often made to feel guilty or responsible for their behavior? Do they monitor or limit your activities, friendships, or access to resources?		
Isolation from support systems	Has your spouse isolated you from your family, friends, or other sources of support? Are you discouraged or prevented from maintaining relationships outside of the marriage? Do you feel socially isolated or dependent solely on your spouse for emotional support?		
Gaslighting	Does your spouse manipulate your perception of reality? Do they deny or minimize their hurtful behavior, making you question your own sanity or memory? Do they frequently twist facts or engage in psychological games to make you doubt your own perceptions?		
Emotional blackmail	Does your spouse use threats or emotional manipulation to control your actions? Do they frequently make ultimatums or withhold love, affection, or support as a means of getting what		

	they want? Do you feel obligated to comply with their demands to avoid negative consequences?		
Intense mood swings or emotional volatility	Does your spouse exhibit extreme mood swings or emotional outbursts? Are you constantly walking on eggshells, trying to avoid triggering their anger or emotional instability? Do you feel responsible for managing their emotions to maintain peace in the relationship?		
Verbal aggression and humiliation:	Does your spouse engage in frequent yelling, shouting, or aggressive language towards you? Do they humiliate or embarrass you, either in private or in front of others? Are you often subjected to insults, name-calling, or derogatory comments?		
Blaming and shifting responsibility	Does your spouse consistently blame you for their own mistakes or shortcomings? Do they avoid taking responsibility for their actions, instead making you feel at fault for their behavior or circumstances?		

Conclusion

As we conclude this chapter, it is essential to remember that emotional abuse is a serious matter that requires recognition and intervention. By understanding the tests, signs, and utilizing an emotional abuse checklist, individuals can begin to unravel the complexities of their relationships and take steps toward healing. In the next chapter, we will delve deeper into the psychological impact of emotional abuse, exploring its long-term effects and avenues for recovery. Remember, you are not alone, and there is hope for a life free from emotional abuse.

Chapter Summary

•   Emotional abuse is a destructive form of mistreatment that can leave lasting scars on one's emotional well-being.

•   Understanding emotional abuse requires evaluating relationships through tests, recognizing common signs, and using an emotional abuse checklist.

•   Five common signs of emotional abuse include constant criticism and belittlement, manipulation and control, isolation from support systems, gaslighting, and emotional blackmail. These signs erode self-esteem, create dependency, undermine reality, and instill fear and guilt.

An emotional abuse checklist provides a comprehensive tool to assess the health of relationships, including dimensions such as verbal aggression, social isolation, financial control, and psychological manipulation.

Chapter 4: Circles and cycles

In the shadows of seemingly perfect relationships lie the haunting truths of emotional abuse. Brace yourself, for within these pages, we shall unravel the chilling reality of the Five Cycles of Emotional Abuse [8].

In this chapter, we delve deep into the complex and often misunderstood realm of emotional abuse. While physical abuse leaves visible scars, emotional abuse can inflict wounds that remain hidden, yet can be equally devastating. By shedding light on the Five Cycles of Emotional Abuse, we aim to provide a comprehensive understanding of this toxic dynamic. Each cycle represents a distinct pattern of behavior that perpetrators employ to manipulate and control their victims, causing immense psychological harm. Through the use of real-life examples and compelling stories, we will explore these cycles in detail, offering insights and awareness to help break the cycle of abuse.

Cycle 1: Disparagement and Demeaning

The first cycle begins with the gradual erosion of a victim's self-esteem through constant disparagement and demeaning remarks. Perpetrators may use insults, criticism, and humiliation as weapons, effectively diminishing their partner's self-worth.

I will illustrate this first cycle using a case I dealt with a few years ago. Elsa was once a vibrant and confident woman, with a contagious smile that lit up the room. She possessed an unwavering belief in herself and her abilities, radiating a sense of purpose and strength. However, her life took a sinister turn when she met Jason, a charming and charismatic man who hid his true colors beneath a veil of charisma.

In the early days of their relationship, Jason seemed like the perfect partner. He showered Elsa with compliments, painting an idyllic picture of their future together. Little did she know that beneath his honeyed words lay a malevolent intent.

The insults began subtly, like venomous whispers in Elsa's ear. At first, they seemed like harmless critiques disguised as jokes. Jason would make offhand comments about her appearance, belittling her in front of others with veiled sarcasm. Elsa laughed nervously, brushing off the subtle digs, convinced they were harmless quirks in an otherwise loving relationship.

But as time went on, Jason's insults grew bolder, striking at the very core of Elsa's self-esteem. He meticulously chipped away at her confidence, leaving her emotionally wounded and questioning her worth. Each cutting remark pierced her like a dagger, causing her spirit to wither and her inner light to fade.

Day by day, Elsa's once vibrant personality retreated further into the shadows. She began to doubt herself, believing every cruel word that Jason uttered. Her reflection in the mirror became distorted, morphing into a distorted image of inadequacy. She no longer recognized the woman staring back at her, as she had become a mere shadow of her former self.

As her confidence eroded, Elsa found herself becoming increasingly dependent on Jason. She clung to him like a lifeline, desperately seeking validation and approval. He had become the sole arbiter of her self-worth, and she became trapped in a web of emotional dependency.

Elsa's friends and family grew concerned, noticing the drastic change in her demeanor. They saw a once vibrant woman reduced to a mere shell, tiptoeing around Jason's volatile moods, afraid of setting off another storm of insults. They tried to intervene, urging her to leave the toxic relationship, but Elsa was ensnared in the illusion that Jason had created.

In moments of solitude, Elsa would reminisce about the confident woman she used to be. She yearned for the strength to break free from Jason's toxic grip, to reclaim her shattered identity. But the scars of emotional abuse ran deep, intertwining with her very sense of self. The thought of leaving terrified her, as she doubted her ability to survive on her own.

However, a glimmer of hope flickered within Elsa's heart. With each insult, a tiny ember of resilience ignited within her. She started to question the narrative that Jason had woven around her, recognizing the insidious manipulation for what it was. In the midst of her darkest moments, she found solace in the realization that she deserved better.

With newfound determination, Elsa began the long and arduous journey toward healing. She sought therapy from us, surrounding herself with a support network that uplifted and believed in her. Slowly but surely, she started to rebuild her shattered confidence, piece by fragile piece.

Elsa's story informs us that emotional abuse can leave scars that are invisible to the naked eye but devastatingly real to the victim. It highlights the insidious nature of relentless insults and their ability to dismantle even the strongest of individuals. Yet, within the depths of despair, the human spirit has the power to rise, to reclaim its true essence and defy the darkness that once consumed it.

Cycle 2: Isolation and Alienation Isolation and alienation

 mark the second cycle, where perpetrators aim to isolate their victims from their support systems, friends, and family. By cutting off these crucial connections, they gain full control over their partner's emotions and actions.

We explore the case of James, whose wife systematically isolated him from his loved ones, leaving him utterly dependent on her, further intensifying her control. In a quaint suburban neighborhood, James and his wife, Emma, appeared to be the picture-perfect couple. Behind closed doors, however, their relationship hid a sinister secret. James's life took an unexpected turn as he became entangled in a web of isolation meticulously woven by Emma, ensnaring him in a labyrinth of emotional dependence.

When James and Emma first met, their love was undeniable. They were inseparable, basking in the euphoria of new romance. Emma, a master of manipulation, recognized James's close bond with his friends and family as a potential threat to her control. With a deceptive smile, she began her insidious campaign to isolate him.

At first, Emma's tactics were subtle. She would express concern about James spending too much time with his friends, subtly planting seeds of doubt in his mind. She would casually mention how his loved ones didn't truly understand their relationship, undermining the strength of his support system. James, blinded by love, failed to recognize the calculated nature of Emma's actions.

As time went on, Emma's methods grew more overt. She would find ways to subtly sabotage his plans to meet friends or attend family gatherings, using manipulation and guilt to keep him within her grasp. Emma's ultimate goal was to sever James's connections, ensuring that he would have no choice but to rely solely on her for companionship, validation, and emotional support.

Gradually, the once-vibrant tapestry of James's social life began to unravel. Friends who once filled his days with laughter and camaraderie were slowly pushed to the periphery of his existence. Emma orchestrated a systematic withdrawal from his loved ones, isolating him from the relationships that had nourished his soul for so long.

As the web of isolation tightened around him, James found

himself increasingly dependent on Emma for emotional sustenance. She became his sole confidante, his only source of comfort in a world that seemed to shrink with every passing day. He no longer had the laughter of friends or the embrace of family to provide solace during difficult times. Emma had effectively become his emotional lifeline, and he clung to her with desperation.

James's isolation was both physical and emotional. Emma's manipulative tactics extended beyond limiting his interactions with others. She also isolated him from the outside world, controlling his access to information and restricting his freedom. She monitored his phone calls, scrutinized his messages, and even limited his access to social media. Emma's hold on James tightened, suffocating his sense of autonomy and leaving him feeling trapped within the confines of their relationship.

The outside world became a distant memory for James. The once vibrant streets were replaced with the suffocating silence of their home. Each day became a monotonous routine, revolving solely around Emma's desires and whims. James yearned for connection, for the warmth of human interaction, but Emma had ensured that he was marooned on an emotional island.

But even within the darkest corners of isolation, a flicker of resilience can ignite. James's spirit refused to be extinguished completely. A chance encounter with an old friend, whom Emma had managed to keep hidden from him, sparked a glimmer of hope. In that brief interaction, James felt a renewed sense of his true self, a reminder of the person he had been before the web of isolation had ensnared him.

With newfound determination, James sought solace in the few remaining fragments of his support system. He confided in his trusted friend, sharing the suffocating reality of his isolation. Together, they devised a plan to liberate James from Emma's clutches and restore his freedom.

It was a risky endeavor, filled with uncertainty and fear, but James summoned his strength and confronted Emma. The web of isolation, once unbreakable, began to unravel as James reclaimed his voice and his connections. With the support of his loved ones, he gradually rebuilt the bridges that had been burned, rediscovering the power of genuine relationships that had sustained him in the past.

James's story demonstrates the insidious nature of isolation and the power it holds to intensify control within an abusive relationship. It serves as a reminder that no one should be held captive by emotional dependence, and that true freedom lies in forging connections that nourish the soul. James's journey is a beacon of hope, a testament to the resilience of the human spirit, and a reminder that even the most intricate web of isolation can be unraveled, setting one free to embrace the world once more.

Cycle 3: Gaslighting and Manipulation

The third cycle introduces gaslighting and manipulation, where perpetrators distort reality, making their victims question their own sanity. Through lies, manipulation, and emotional blackmail, they sow doubt and confusion, weakening their partner's grasp on reality.

Emily's journey illustrates the insidious effects of gaslighting, as her husband systematically manipulated her perceptions, leading her to question her own judgment. Emily and her husband, Mark, led a pretty envious life having met in the university and went on to get married in a big church ceremony. Yet, beneath the illusion of happiness lay a twisted game of manipulation and deceit. Emily's journey unraveled the chilling effects of gaslighting, as Mark orchestrated a psychological maze, leaving her questioning her sanity and reality itself.

Their relationship began with promises of eternal love and unwavering support. Mark, a master puppeteer, skillfully wove his web of deception, preying upon Emily's vulnerabilities and deepest fears. He knew exactly which strings to pull to gain control over her mind and emotions.

At first, Mark's manipulation was subtle. He would make sly comments that subtly contradicted Emily's perceptions, leaving her with a lingering sense of doubt. He would undermine her memories of past events, dismissing her recollections as faulty and unreliable. Over time, these small seeds of doubt grew into a dense forest of confusion within Emily's mind.

Mark's gaslighting tactics escalated gradually, like a symphony of deception carefully orchestrated to erode Emily's sense of reality. He would rearrange objects in their home, subtly moving them out of place, only to deny any involvement when Emily questioned the changes. He would insist that conversations they had never occurred, causing Emily to question her own sanity.

As Mark's manipulation deepened, he skillfully distorted the truth to fit his own narrative. He would twist Emily's words, manipulating their meaning to make her doubt her intentions and motives. He strategically undermined her self-confidence, subtly chipping away at her self-esteem, until she became an obedient puppet in his intricate game of control.

Emily's mind became a battleground of conflicting thoughts and emotions. She questioned her own judgment, doubting her perception of reality. Gaslighting left her feeling disoriented and emotionally fragile, as if she were living in a distorted version of the world she once knew. Her sense of self began to crumble, leaving her teetering on the precipice of a psychological abyss.

As the web of gaslighting tightened its grip, Emily's support system dwindled. Mark had systematically alienated her from friends and family, leaving her alone and vulnerable to his manipulation. She had no one to turn to, no external validation to counter the gaslighting that had become her reality.

But deep within Emily's soul, a spark of resilience flickered. She refused to surrender her sanity to Mark's gaslighting game. With unwavering determination, she embarked on a journey of self-discovery, seeking out therapy and support groups where she could share her experiences.

In the safe space of these support networks, Emily encountered others who had endured similar manipulations. Their stories, filled with courage and resilience, became beacons of hope that illuminated her path towards healing. Together, they unraveled the intricate web of gaslighting, exposing its insidious nature and reclaiming their truths.

As Emily gained clarity, her confidence soared. She learned to trust her instincts again, rebuilding the fractured pieces of her identity that Mark had shattered. She confronted his gaslighting tactics head-on, refusing to let his lies define her reality any longer.

Emily's journey serves as a haunting reminder of the devastating impact of gaslighting. It sheds light on the profound effects of psychological manipulation and the dangerous power it holds to distort one's perception of reality. Her story stands as a testament to the indomitable spirit that can emerge from the darkest depths, as she rediscovered her strength and reclaimed her truth, breaking free from the shadows of deception that had once entrapped her.

Cycle 4: Emotional Withholding and Neglect Emotional

withholding and neglect characterize the fourth cycle, wherein the abuser deprives their partner of emotional support, validation, and intimacy. They withhold affection, empathy, and attention, leaving the victim starved for emotional nourishment.

Jack's experience highlights the profound impact of emotional neglect, as his wife consistently denied him the love and care he craved, leaving him feeling empty and unimportant. In a quiet suburban neighborhood, Jack's life unfolded with a deafening silence. His story reveals the profound impact of emotional neglect, as his wife, Lily, erected an impenetrable wall between them, denying him the love and care he craved. Day by day, Jack's spirit withered as he was left feeling empty, unimportant, and invisible.

When Jack and Lily first embarked on their journey together, there was a glimmer of hope. They shared dreams, aspirations, and promises of a fulfilling life. However, as time passed, Lily's true nature revealed itself—an emotional void that consumed her, leaving Jack stranded in a desolate landscape of neglect.

Emotional neglect can be a subtle and insidious form of abuse. It is the absence of emotional attunement, support, and genuine connection that chips away at a person's soul. In Jack's case, Lily's emotional neglect manifested as an impassable chasm that separated them, leaving him standing on the edge of an abyss of loneliness.

Lily consistently withheld the affection and care that Jack yearned for. She dismissed his emotional needs, minimizing their importance, and leaving him feeling insignificant. Her indifference towards his pain eroded the foundation of their relationship, one neglected emotion at a time.

Jack's attempts to bridge the emotional gap were met with indifference or even contempt. He longed for heartfelt conversations and gestures of love, but his pleas fell on deaf ears. Lily's emotional absence left Jack feeling like an empty vessel, desperately seeking fulfillment but continually met with disappointment.

The void within Jack grew wider with each passing day. He questioned his worth, wondering why he couldn't elicit the love and attention he so desperately desired. His self-esteem plummeted as he internalized Lily's emotional neglect, believing he was undeserving of love and affection.

Jack's world became a desolate landscape, devoid of color and warmth. The laughter and joy that once filled their home were replaced by an eerie silence. The emptiness gnawed at his core, leaving him emotionally starved and gasping for the nourishment of genuine connection.

To cope with the pain, Jack tried to bury his emotions, building walls around his heart to protect himself from further hurt. Yet, the numbness that enveloped him was a constant reminder of the love and care he craved but could never attain. His soul yearned for the intimacy that had been cruelly denied, leaving him perpetually adrift in a sea of emotional emptiness.

But deep within Jack's desolation, a flicker of self-compassion emerged. He began to recognize that the void within him was not a reflection of his inherent worth, but a consequence of Lily's emotional neglect. He sought solace in therapy, where he discovered that he was deserving of love, care, and emotional nourishment.

With support from his therapist, Jack embarked on a journey of self-discovery and healing. He learned to validate his own emotions and embrace his needs, dismantling the belief that he was unworthy of love. Through self-reflection and self-care, he gradually rebuilt his shattered self-esteem, finding the strength to redefine his understanding of love and seek out healthier relationships.

Jack's odyssey highlights the profound impact of emotional neglect on one's psyche. It serves as a reminder of the importance of emotional attunement, empathy, and genuine connection in any relationship. Jack's story encourages us to recognize the damaging effects of neglect and to strive for relationships that nurture our emotional well-being, ensuring that no one is left drowning in the depths of emotional emptiness.

Cycle 5: Escalation and Explosions

The fifth cycle, escalation and explosions, represents the culmination of emotional abuse, marked by explosive outbursts of anger, rage, and aggression. Perpetrators unleash their pent-up emotions, using fear and intimidation to maintain control over their partners.

Tanisha's story serves as a chilling reminder of the devastating consequences of such explosive behavior, as her partner's rage escalated to physical violence, forever changing her life. Tanisha 's life took a dark and harrowing turn as her partner's rage escalated from verbal abuse to physical violence. The echoes of pain reverberated through her soul, forever changing her life and leaving an indelible mark on her child's innocent world.

Tanisha 's tale began like any other love story. She believed she had found her knight in shining armor, a man who would protect and cherish her. However, beneath his charming façade lurked a volatile temperament, ready to unleash a storm of anger and aggression at a moment's notice.

The cracks in their relationship became apparent as her

partner's outbursts intensified. Initially, his anger manifested in verbal assaults, hurling insults that cut to the core of Tanisha 's self-worth. He manipulated her emotions, playing on her vulnerabilities to maintain control. Each tirade left Tanisha questioning her worth, her spirit slowly eroding with every toxic word.

As time passed, her partner's explosive behavior escalated to physical violence. The once tender and loving home transformed into a battlefield, where Tanisha bore the brunt of his uncontrollable rage. The world around her became a blur of fear and pain, as she desperately sought refuge from the storm of violence that engulfed her life.

Tanisha 's love for her child added an agonizing layer to her suffering. With each act of violence, her heart broke not only for herself but for the innocent eyes that witnessed the horrors inflicted upon their mother. The weight of responsibility to protect her child clashed with the fear that paralyzed her, creating a suffocating sense of helplessness.

In the shadows of the night, Tanisha 's resilience flickered. She found solace in the support of a domestic violence hotline, a lifeline that provided her with the resources and courage to break free from the cycle of abuse. With their guidance, she orchestrated a plan to escape, her determination fueled by the love she had for her child and a desperate yearning for a life free from violence.

Leaving her abuser behind was no easy feat. It meant uprooting her life, severing ties with toxic relationships, and rebuilding from the shattered fragments of her existence. But Tanisha 's courage knew no bounds, and she navigated the treacherous path toward freedom with unwavering determination.

As she began her healing journey, Tanisha sought refuge in therapy from my office and support groups that I connected her with. The scars, both visible and invisible, became markers of her resilience and a testament to the strength that had propelled her forward. Through the support of compassionate professionals and fellow survivors, Tanisha learned to reclaim her power, redefining her identity beyond the confines of the abuse she had endured.

Tanisha 's story shows the far-reaching consequences of explosive behavior within intimate relationships. It underscores the urgent need for societal awareness and support systems that empower survivors and hold perpetrators accountable. Her tale ignites a call to action, urging us to break the silence and dismantle the systems that perpetuate the cycle of violence.

As Tanisha continues to rebuild her life, her child's innocence is slowly restored. The echoes of pain are replaced by whispers of hope, as they embark on a new chapter filled with love, safety, and the unwavering belief that they deserve a future free from the shadows of abuse.

Conclusion

The Five Cycles of Emotional Abuse provide a framework for understanding the intricacies of emotional abuse within relationships. By examining each cycle and the accompanying examples and stories, we hope to equip individuals with the knowledge and awareness needed to recognize and address emotional abuse. It is crucial to break the silence surrounding this pervasive issue and empower survivors to seek help, rebuild their lives, and foster healthy, loving relationships.

Remember, the journey to healing begins with acknowledging the darkness, and together we can illuminate the path towards a brighter future, free from the shackles of emotional abuse.

Summary

Here are the five points summarizing the Five Cycles of Emotional Abuse:

- Cycle 1: Disparagement and Demeaning - Perpetrators erode the victim's self-esteem through constant criticism, insults, and humiliation, diminishing their self-worth.

- Cycle 2: Isolation and Alienation - Perpetrators isolate victims from their support systems, friends, and family, gaining full control over their emotions and actions.

- Cycle 3: Gaslighting and Manipulation - Perpetrators distort reality, making victims question their own sanity through lies, manipulation, and emotional blackmail.

- Cycle 4: Emotional Withholding and Neglect - Perpetrators deprive victims of emotional support, validation, and intimacy, withholding affection, empathy, and attention.

- Cycle 5: Intermittent Rewards and Punishments - Perpetrators alternate between moments of kindness and cruelty, keeping victims emotionally invested and dependent on their unpredictable behavior.

These cycles represent distinct patterns of behavior that emotional abusers employ to manipulate and control their victims, causing psychological harm. Understanding these cycles can help raise awareness and break the cycle of abuse.

Chapter 5: Get up, go on

"Out of suffering have emerged the strongest souls; the most massive characters are seared with scars." - Kahlil Gibran

In the journey of healing from emotional abuse, individuals often undergo a series of phases that lead them towards reclaiming their power, finding inner strength, and rebuilding their lives. These phases are not linear, and the progression through them can vary from person to person. However, understanding the common patterns can provide valuable insights and guidance for survivors and those who support them. This chapter explores the six phases of healing from emotional abuse [9], drawing upon various psychological theories and providing practical examples of how these phases can be applied.

Phase 1: Awareness and Acknowledgment

The first phase of healing involves becoming aware of the emotional abuse and acknowledging its impact. This phase aligns with the cognitive-behavioral theory, which emphasizes the role of thoughts and beliefs in shaping emotions and behaviors. By recognizing the abusive patterns, survivors can challenge the distorted beliefs instilled by the abuser and begin to reclaim their sense of self.

"Remember, you have been criticizing yourself for years and it hasn't worked. Try approving of yourself and see what happens." - Louise Hay

In the aftermath of emotional abuse, survivors often grapple with a distorted sense of self-worth, deeply influenced by the constant criticism and belittlement they endured. However, as survivors embark on their healing journey, they gradually come to the profound realization that the relentless criticism was not a reflection of their inherent worth, but rather a manipulative tactic employed by the abuser to gain control over them.

Let's delve into two personal stories that illustrate this transformative realization:

Samantha's Story: Samantha had spent years trapped in an emotionally abusive relationship. Her partner consistently criticized her appearance, intelligence, and abilities, eroding her self-esteem and leaving her feeling worthless. The impact of the constant criticism was deeply ingrained in Samantha's psyche, leading her to question her own worth and capabilities long after she escaped the abusive relationship.

However, as Samantha began her healing process, she

sought therapy with a compassionate counselor who helped her gain insight into the dynamics of emotional abuse. Through therapy, she began to understand that the relentless criticism was not a reflection of her true worth, but rather a manipulative tool used by her abuser to maintain power and control over her.

With this newfound awareness, Samantha gradually detached herself from the harmful narratives instilled by her abuser. She learned to challenge the negative self-talk that had been deeply ingrained in her mind and replace it with affirmations of her inherent worth and value. Samantha started embracing her unique qualities and talents, recognizing that the constant criticism had been a tactic to diminish her confidence and keep her under the abuser's control. Through self-compassion and support from therapy, Samantha reclaimed her sense of self-worth and began to rebuild her life on a foundation of self-love and empowerment.

Michael's Story: Michael had grown up in a household where emotional abuse was prevalent. His parents consistently criticized his every move, undermining his confidence and devaluing his accomplishments. As a result, Michael internalized the criticism, viewing himself as inherently flawed and unworthy of love and acceptance.

It wasn't until Michael sought support from a support group for survivors of emotional abuse that he began to challenge his deeply ingrained belief system. In the group, he listened to stories of fellow survivors and realized that the criticism he endured was not a reflection of his true worth but rather a manipulation tactic used by his parents to exert control.

Inspired by the collective strength of the support group, Michael started engaging in self-reflection and self-compassion practices. He began to separate his sense of self-worth from the toxic narratives he had internalized. Through therapy and personal growth work, Michael learned to recognize his strengths, accomplishments, and unique qualities. He acknowledged that the constant criticism he faced in his childhood had been a tactic to maintain power and control, and it did not define his true value as an individual.

With this newfound perspective, Michael gradually shed the weight of self-doubt and embraced his inherent worth. He embarked on a journey of self-discovery, pursuing his passions, setting boundaries, and surrounding himself with supportive and nurturing relationships. Through his healing process, Michael became an advocate for survivors of emotional abuse, sharing his story and empowering others to break free from the damaging effects of constant criticism.

These personal stories demonstrate the transformative realization that the constant criticism survivors endured during emotional abuse was not a reflection of their worth. It was a manipulative tactic employed by abusers to gain control. Through self-reflection, therapy, and support from others, survivors can dismantle the damaging narratives and rebuild their self-worth based on their inherent value as individuals. As survivors embrace this profound realization, they embark on a path of healing, self-acceptance, and empowerment.

Phase 2: Self-Care and Boundaries

In this phase, survivors focus on self-care and establishing healthy boundaries. This aligns with the attachment theory, which highlights the importance of secure relationships and self-regulation. By prioritizing their well-being, survivors learn to nurture themselves and develop a strong support network. Setting boundaries becomes crucial in preventing further abuse and creating a safe environment.

Emotional abuse survivors often learn to say no to unreasonable demands and prioritize their own needs without guilt or fear. For instance, Lily who had spent years trapped in an emotionally abusive marriage, took steps to break free from the chains that had entangled her. Her partner constantly belittled her, controlled her every move, and demanded her unwavering obedience. Under the weight of his unreasonable demands, Lily had lost sight of her own needs and desires, catering solely to the whims of her abusive partner.

However, one fateful day, Lily summoned the courage to break free from the toxic relationship. As she embarked on her journey of healing, she discovered the transformative power of setting boundaries and prioritizing her own needs without guilt or fear.

Lily's newfound determination led her to seek therapy with a compassionate counselor who specialized in trauma recovery. In the safe and non-judgmental space of therapy, Lily began to unravel the layers of conditioning and self-doubt instilled by her abuser. Through introspection and guidance from her therapist, she gradually realized that her worth was not defined by her ability to meet unreasonable demands, but rather by her inherent value as a human being.

Armed with this newfound understanding, Lily embarked on the challenging path of asserting her boundaries and prioritizing her needs. She learned to say "no" to unreasonable demands and toxic situations that compromised her well-being. At first, guilt and fear threatened to hold her back, as remnants of her past conditioning whispered in her mind, reminding her of the consequences she had faced for resisting her abuser's control.

But Lily refused to be silenced any longer. She recognized that her needs and happiness were equally valid and deserving of attention. Drawing strength from therapy, support groups, and the stories of other survivors, she began to reclaim her voice and assert her boundaries with unwavering determination.

There were times when Lily's abuser, sensing his loss of control, attempted to manipulate her into surrendering to his demands once again. But Lily stood firm, armed with the knowledge that her well-being and self-respect were paramount. She reminded herself that she deserved to be treated with respect and dignity.

Over time, Lily's courage and unwavering commitment to her own needs began to yield profound changes in her life. She noticed that as she set and maintained boundaries, the people around her began to respect and honor her wishes. Her relationships with friends and family deepened, as they witnessed her newfound assertiveness and supported her in her journey of healing.

Through her experiences, Lily became an inspiration for others who had endured emotional abuse. She joined support groups and advocacy organizations, sharing her story and empowering fellow survivors to embrace their own worth and assert their boundaries. Lily's transformation and resilience demonstrated that it was possible to break free from the chains of emotional abuse, reclaim one's voice, and prioritize personal needs without guilt or fear.

In learning to say no to unreasonable demands and prioritizing her own needs, Lily discovered a newfound freedom and self-empowerment. Her journey affirms that survivors of emotional abuse can protect themselves, set boundaries, and prioritize their well-being without guilt or fear.

Phase 3: Processing and Grieving

During this phase, survivors process the emotional pain and grieve the losses they experienced. This phase aligns with the stages of grief proposed by Elisabeth Kübler-Ross, which include denial, anger, bargaining, depression, and acceptance [10]. Survivors may go through these stages repeatedly as they confront the magnitude of their experiences. Through therapy, support groups, or journaling, survivors can navigate their emotions and gradually find healing.

A survivor may feel anger towards the abuser for the injustice they endured, followed by moments of sadness and finally, acceptance that the abuse was not their fault.

To understand this phase, let's look at a real-life story. Chelsea, a vibrant and ambitious woman, found herself trapped in a toxic relationship with a manipulative partner named Ed. Throughout their time together, Ed constantly belittled Chelsea, undermined her self-esteem, and controlled her every move. The emotional abuse she endured left deep scars on her psyche, causing her to question her worth and blame herself for the mistreatment.

At first, Chelsea 's overwhelming emotion was anger. She felt a righteous fury towards Ed for subjecting her to such unjust treatment. This anger fueled her determination to break free from the toxic cycle and regain control over her life. Chelsea sought support from friends, family, and therapy, which empowered her to recognize the abuse for what it truly was.

However, beneath the surface anger lay a profound sadness. Chelsea mourned the loss of the relationship she had once believed in, grieving for the dreams and hopes that had been shattered by the emotional abuse. The realization that someone she loved and trusted had betrayed her confidence deeply wounded her. She struggled with feelings of loneliness, betrayal, and heartache, often questioning why she had allowed herself to endure such mistreatment.

As time passed, Chelsea gradually began to embrace the third stage of her journey: acceptance. Through therapy and self-reflection, she came to understand that the abuse was never her fault. She recognized that the abuser's actions were a reflection of his own insecurities and control issues, rather than any deficiency on her part. Chelsea acknowledged that she deserved love, respect, and kindness, just like anyone else.

Acceptance did not mean forgetting or condoning the abuse, but rather liberating herself from the burden of blame. Chelsea let go of the toxic emotions that had weighed her down, forgiving herself for any perceived shortcomings and acknowledging her own strength and resilience. She focused on rebuilding her life, rediscovering her passions, and cultivating healthier relationships.

Chelsea 's story serves as a powerful example of the journey that survivors of emotional abuse often embark upon. It highlights the range of emotions they experience, from anger and sadness to eventual acceptance. It also underscores the importance of seeking support, therapy, and self-reflection to heal from the wounds inflicted by emotional abuse. Chelsea 's transformation from a survivor to a thriver is a testament to the human spirit's capacity to heal, grow, and find peace after enduring such profound injustice.

Phase 4: Rebuilding Self-Esteem and Identity

In this phase, survivors work on rebuilding their self-esteem and redefining their identity. This aligns with the humanistic theory, which emphasizes self-actualization and personal growth. Survivors explore their strengths, values, and interests, rekindling their passions and discovering new aspects of themselves. By engaging in self-reflection and embracing their authenticity, survivors can restore their sense of self-worth.

As survivors of emotional abuse embark on their healing journey, a crucial phase involves rebuilding themselves and rediscovering their sense of joy, purpose, and personal fulfillment. This phase is marked by engaging in activities that bring them genuine happiness, pursuing new hobbies or interests, and rekindling long-lost dreams. These endeavors not only promote self-discovery but also play a vital role in reclaiming one's identity and fostering a sense of empowerment.

For example, let's consider the story of Alex, a survivor who endured years of emotional abuse in a toxic work environment. Throughout this traumatic period, Alex's passion for painting, which had once brought them immense joy, was overshadowed and ultimately abandoned due to the constant criticism and belittling from their colleagues and supervisors. However, as Alex embarked on their healing journey, they recognized the importance of reconnecting with their creative side as a means of reclaiming their identity and finding joy once again.

With the support of therapy and a strong network of friends, Alex began to allocate time to engage in painting activities. They joined local art classes and workshops, surrounded themselves with like-minded individuals who shared their passion, and gradually rediscovered the therapeutic and empowering nature of art. Painting became a cathartic outlet for Alex to express their emotions, process their experiences, and regain a sense of control over their life.

In addition to rekindling their artistic pursuits, survivors often explore new hobbies and interests that align with their authentic selves. For instance, Liz, another survivor of emotional abuse, had always been intrigued by the world of gardening but had never given herself the opportunity to indulge in this passion. During her healing process, Liz decided to transform her backyard into a small garden sanctuary. She immersed herself in learning about plants, gardening techniques, and sustainable practices. As Liz watched her garden flourish, she found solace in the nurturing process, gained a sense of accomplishment, and experienced a profound connection with nature. Engaging in this new hobby allowed her to cultivate a renewed sense of purpose and delight in the simple joys of tending to her plants and witnessing their growth.

Survivors also often revisit long-lost dreams or aspirations that were overshadowed or discouraged during the abusive relationship. Let's consider the story of Mark, a survivor who had always dreamt of writing a novel but was repeatedly undermined and told that his writing was insignificant by his abusive partner. Following his escape from the toxic relationship, Mark decided to reignite his passion for storytelling. He enrolled in writing courses, joined a local writing group, and dedicated time each day to work on his novel. Through this creative process, Mark not only rediscovered his love for writing but also gained a newfound sense of purpose and accomplishment. As he completed his novel and shared his story with others, he found validation, support, and a sense of achievement, empowering him to embrace his identity as a writer.

Engaging in activities that bring joy, pursuing new hobbies, or reconnecting with long-lost dreams serve as powerful tools for survivors to rebuild themselves and reclaim their sense of identity and purpose. These endeavors provide avenues for self-expression, personal growth, and the cultivation of joy and fulfillment. Through these transformative experiences, survivors not only rediscover their passions but also forge a path towards healing, self-empowerment, and a renewed zest for life.

Phase 5: Developing Healthy Relationships During this phase, survivors learn to develop healthy relationships based on trust, respect, and mutual support. This aligns with the social cognitive theory, which emphasizes the reciprocal influence between individuals and their social environment. Survivors work on enhancing their communication skills, setting healthy boundaries, and identifying red flags in relationships. By surrounding themselves with positive influences, survivors can create a supportive network that fosters their healing.

After enduring the trauma of emotional abuse, survivors often recognize the crucial role of healthy relationships in their healing journey. In their efforts to rebuild their lives, survivors may intentionally cultivate friendships with individuals who value and uplift them, or they may seek therapy to develop healthier relationship patterns. These actions contribute to the creation of a support network that fosters healing, self-worth, and the cultivation of positive connections.

Consider the story of Emily, a survivor who had been subjected to years of emotional abuse within her family. As Emily began her healing process, she realized the significance of surrounding herself with individuals who genuinely cared for her well-being. She sought out friendships that were based on trust, respect, and mutual support. Emily made a conscious effort to connect with people who valued her for who she truly was, rather than perpetuating the cycle of toxic relationships that had defined her past.

One day, Emily attended a local support group for survivors of emotional abuse. It was there that she met Rachel, another survivor who shared similar experiences. They immediately connected on a deep level, understanding each other's pain and journey towards healing. Emily and Rachel formed a strong bond, providing each other with empathy, encouragement, and a safe space to share their stories without judgment. Through their friendship, Emily found solace in knowing that she was not alone in her struggles and that she had someone who genuinely understood and supported her.

Alongside cultivating friendships, survivors may also choose to seek therapy to address the psychological and emotional wounds inflicted by emotional abuse. Therapy provides a structured and professional environment where survivors can explore their experiences, process their emotions, and develop healthier relationship patterns. With the guidance of a therapist, survivors gain insight into the dynamics of abusive relationships, learn to recognize and challenge negative patterns, and acquire essential skills for setting boundaries and establishing healthy connections.

Returning to Emily's story, after months of reflection and introspection, she decided to seek therapy to aid her healing process further. In therapy, Emily worked with a compassionate and trauma-informed therapist who specialized in helping survivors of emotional abuse. Through their sessions, Emily unpacked the deep-rooted beliefs instilled by the abuse, addressed her emotional wounds, and developed strategies to cultivate healthier relationship patterns.

With time and the support of her therapist, Emily gained a stronger sense of self-worth and a clearer understanding of what healthy relationships entailed. She learned to set boundaries, communicate her needs effectively, and recognize red flags in potential relationships. Emily's therapy journey not only facilitated her healing but also provided her with a solid foundation to build and sustain healthy connections in her personal and professional life.

By deliberately cultivating friendships with individuals who uplifted her and seeking therapy to develop healthier relationship patterns, Emily took significant steps towards rebuilding her life after emotional abuse. Through these intentional actions, she created a support network that nurtured her healing process, promoted self-worth, and fostered the growth of positive, empowering relationships.

In the journey of healing from emotional abuse, the cultivation of healthy relationships and the exploration of therapeutic interventions serve as crucial pillars of support. These intentional steps help survivors reframe their understanding of relationships, develop healthy attachment patterns, and surround themselves with individuals who contribute positively to their well-being. Ultimately, these actions contribute to the restoration of their self-esteem, the reconstruction of their social support network, and the establishment of healthier, more fulfilling connections.

Phase 6: Integration and Post-Traumatic Growth

In the final phase, survivors integrate their healing journey into their lives and experience post-traumatic growth. This aligns with the concept of post-traumatic growth, which suggests that individuals can grow stronger and find meaning in the aftermath of trauma. Survivors recognize the wisdom and resilience gained from their experiences and use it as a catalyst for personal transformation. They may channel their healing into helping others, engaging in advocacy work, or pursuing meaningful goals.

Survivors of emotional abuse often find tremendous strength in sharing their stories and advocating for others who have endured similar experiences. By speaking out, they not only raise awareness about the devastating effects of emotional abuse but also provide support, validation, and hope to fellow survivors. Additionally, their advocacy efforts can inspire change in societal attitudes, systems, and policies, creating a safer and more compassionate environment for individuals affected by emotional abuse.

One inspiring example of a survivor-turned-advocate is Alice. Alice experienced years of emotional abuse in a toxic relationship, enduring constant belittling, manipulation, and control from her partner. After finding the courage to leave the abusive situation and embark on her healing journey, Alice realized the transformative power of sharing her story. Recognizing that emotional abuse was often misunderstood and overlooked, she felt a deep calling to raise awareness and support others in similar situations.

Alice started by writing a blog where she candidly shared her experiences, emotions, and the challenges she faced during her healing process. Her words resonated with countless readers, many of whom reached out to express gratitude for giving voice to their own hidden pain. Encouraged by the impact her writing had, Alice began attending local support groups for survivors of emotional abuse, where she met others who shared their stories and struggles.

Inspired by the collective strength and determination of these survivors, Alice realized the power of advocacy in effecting change. She joined forces with local organizations dedicated to supporting survivors of abuse and started volunteering her time and expertise. Together, they organized awareness campaigns, workshops, and events to educate the community about emotional abuse and provide resources for those in need.

Alice 's advocacy work expanded beyond her local community as she became involved with national and international organizations focused on combating emotional abuse. She collaborated with experts in the field, contributed to research projects, and participated in conferences and panel discussions to raise awareness among professionals and policymakers. Through her tireless efforts, Alice became a recognized voice in the field, providing insights, guidance, and hope to countless survivors.

Alice's advocacy work did not stop at raising awareness; she also dedicated herself to driving systemic change. She worked alongside legislators and policymakers to push for stricter laws and regulations to protect survivors of emotional abuse. Her personal experiences and the stories shared by fellow survivors became powerful testimonies that influenced legislation and policies addressing emotional abuse within intimate relationships, workplaces, and educational institutions.

Alice's journey from survivor to advocate exemplifies the transformative impact of using one's story to raise awareness and inspire change. Through her courage, resilience, and unwavering commitment, she has not only reclaimed her own power but also made a lasting impact on the lives of countless individuals affected by emotional abuse. Her advocacy efforts have helped dismantle the silence and stigma surrounding emotional abuse while paving the way for a more compassionate and supportive society.

Conclusion

The six phases of healing from emotional abuse provide a roadmap for survivors as they navigate their journey towards recovery and transformation. By understanding how these phases align with various psychological theories and learning from practical examples, survivors and their supporters can gain valuable insights and guidance. Remember, healing is a personal and unique process, but with perseverance and support, survivors can emerge stronger, reclaim their power, and forge a brighter future beyond the scars of emotional abuse.

Summary:

- Healing from emotional abuse involves going through six phases: awareness and acknowledgment, self-care and boundaries, processing and grieving, rebuilding self-esteem and identity, developing healthy relationships, and embracing self-acceptance and empowerment.

- Survivors of emotional abuse need to become aware of the abuse and its impact, challenge distorted beliefs, and reclaim their sense of self-worth.

- Self-care and setting healthy boundaries are crucial for survivors to prioritize their well-being and create a safe environment for themselves.

- Survivors need to process their emotional pain, grieve their losses, and go through stages of denial, anger, bargaining, depression, and acceptance. They can seek therapy, join support groups, or journal to navigate their emotions and find healing.

☐

Chapter 6: Unshackling

"Sometimes walking away has nothing to do with weakness, and everything to do with strength. We walk away not because we want others to realize our worth and value, but because we finally realize our own."- Robert Tew

In this chapter, we delve into the difficult topic of when and how to walk away from an emotionally abusive relationship, particularly when therapy has failed to address the underlying issues. We understand that making the decision to leave can be immensely challenging, but we want to assure you that it is an act of strength and self-preservation. Throughout this chapter, we will discuss signs that therapy may not be effective, explore possible places partners run to escape abusive marriages, offer encouragement for starting afresh, and share real stories of individuals who found the courage to walk away.

When therapy fails to provide the necessary resolution for emotional abuse, it becomes crucial to recognize the limitations of therapeutic interventions. While therapy can be beneficial for many relationship issues, emotional abuse often requires additional measures. Some signs that therapy may not be working include a lack of progress, continued manipulation, or instances where the abusive partner refuses to acknowledge their harmful behavior. It is important to trust your instincts and understand that seeking alternative options is not a failure but a necessary step towards healing.

When contemplating leaving an emotionally abusive relationship, it is essential to have a plan in place. This plan includes identifying safe places to escape to and seeking support from organizations, shelters, or helplines specializing in assisting individuals in abusive situations. These resources can provide the necessary guidance, protection, and emotional support during the transition.

Leaving an abusive marriage can be a frightening prospect, but it also opens the door to a fresh start. We encourage you to embrace the opportunity for personal growth and self-discovery. Starting afresh involves prioritizing self-care, rebuilding self-esteem, and seeking out positive relationships. We want to emphasize that you deserve happiness and a life free from emotional abuse, and it is within your power to create that reality.

Real stories of resilience and empowerment serve as a testament to the strength and courage of survivors. Through these stories, we aim to inspire and encourage individuals who may be facing similar challenges. We will share narratives of individuals who successfully walked away from emotionally abusive relationships, highlighting their journeys, the obstacles they encountered, and the transformations they underwent. These stories will serve as beacons of hope, demonstrating that there is life beyond abuse and that a brighter future awaits those who take the brave step of leaving.

While therapy may not have provided the desired outcome, seeking professional help remains crucial during this transition. There are various therapeutic approaches beyond traditional therapy that can aid in the healing process. Individual counseling, support groups, and trauma-informed therapies can provide the necessary tools and support needed to navigate the complexities of emotional abuse.

Example 1: Jill's Journey to Freedom

Jill endured years of emotional abuse in her marriage, constantly belittled and controlled by her husband. Despite attending therapy together, the abuse persisted, leaving Jill feeling trapped and hopeless. Recognizing that therapy alone was not enough, she reached out to a local women's shelter for support and guidance.

Leaving her abusive marriage was not easy for Jill. She faced numerous obstacles along the way, including fear of her husband's retaliation and the uncertainty of starting a new life. However, with the help of the shelter, she created a safety plan, secured temporary housing, and obtained a restraining order.

During her healing process, Jill actively participated in individual counseling and joined a support group for survivors of emotional abuse. These resources provided her with a safe space to share her experiences, receive validation, and learn coping mechanisms for the trauma she had endured.

Over time, Jill began to rebuild her self-esteem and regain control over her life. She pursued her passions and enrolled in a career development program, which allowed her to gain financial independence. With newfound confidence and support from her newfound community, Jill successfully walked away from her emotionally abusive relationship.

Today, Jill's transformation is evident. She has embraced her freedom and learned to set boundaries in her relationships. She is an advocate for survivors of emotional abuse, sharing her story to inspire others to break free from their own abusive situations. Jill's journey serves as a testament to the resilience and strength of survivors and offers hope to those who may be in similar circumstances.

Example 2: Shawn's Path to Healing

Shawn spent years in an emotionally abusive relationship, constantly subjected to manipulation, gaslighting, and verbal attacks. Despite attending couples therapy with his partner, the abuse persisted, leaving Shawn feeling emotionally drained and isolated. Realizing that therapy was not enough to bring about change, he made the difficult decision to walk away.

Leaving an emotionally abusive relationship was not without its challenges for Shawn. He faced immense guilt and self-doubt, often questioning whether he was overreacting or responsible for the abuse. However, with the support of a close friend and a therapist specializing in trauma, Shawn gradually regained his sense of self-worth and found the strength to break free.

As part of his healing journey, Shawn immersed himself in self-care practices and sought out alternative therapeutic approaches. He explored mindfulness meditation and engaged in art therapy, allowing him to express and process his emotions in a safe and creative way. Through individual counseling, Shawn worked through the trauma of his past relationship, learning to identify red flags and establish healthier boundaries for future relationships.

Shawn's transformation was gradual but profound. He gradually rebuilt his confidence, surrounded himself with a supportive network of friends, and rediscovered his passions and interests. Today, he is thriving in a new relationship that is based on mutual respect and emotional support.

Shawn's story demonstrates the power of self-reflection and the importance of seeking specialized support when therapy alone falls short. By recognizing the signs of emotional abuse and making the courageous decision to leave, Shawn embarked on a journey of healing and personal growth. His story serves as an inspiration to others who may be trapped in emotionally abusive relationships, showing them that there is hope for a brighter future beyond the pain and turmoil.

Conclusion

Walking away from an emotionally abusive relationship after failed therapy is an act of strength and self-preservation. By recognizing the signs that therapy is ineffective, exploring safe places to escape, and seeking support from organizations, individuals can embark on a journey of healing and personal growth. Remember, you are not alone, and there are resources available to support you. Through the real stories shared in this chapter, we hope to inspire and empower you to take the necessary steps towards a life free from emotional abuse.

Summary

1.   Walking away from an emotionally abusive relationship after failed therapy is an act of strength and self-preservation. Recognizing the signs that therapy is ineffective and understanding the limitations of therapeutic interventions is crucial. It is not a failure to seek alternative options but a necessary step towards healing.

2.   When contemplating leaving an emotionally abusive relationship, having a plan in place is essential. This plan includes identifying safe places to escape to and seeking support from organizations, shelters, or helplines specializing in assisting individuals in abusive situations. These resources provide guidance, protection, and emotional support during the transition.

3.   Leaving an abusive marriage opens the door to a fresh start. Embracing the opportunity for personal growth and self-discovery involves prioritizing self-care, rebuilding self-esteem, and seeking out positive relationships. Real stories of resilience and empowerment serve as beacons of hope, showing that life beyond abuse is

possible.

Final thoughts

This book has delved into the complex and deeply impactful subject of emotional abuse, aiming to provide readers with a comprehensive understanding of its various aspects. Throughout the chapters, we have explored the different facets of emotional abuse, from its definition and manifestations to the long-term effects it can have on individuals.

Chapter 1 served as an introduction to emotional abuse, shedding light on what it entails, how it manifests, and why it occurs. By unraveling the dynamics of emotional abuse, readers gained a deeper understanding of the tactics used by abusers and the psychological impact they can have on their victims.

Building upon this foundation, Chapter 2 explored the emotionally abusive mind. By delving into the mindset of abusers, readers gained insight into the underlying motivations and psychological factors that drive their behavior. This chapter aimed to foster empathy while emphasizing the importance of recognizing and addressing abusive tendencies.

Chapter 3 focused on the crucial task of identifying emotional abuse. By equipping readers with knowledge and awareness, the chapter provided tools to recognize the signs and patterns of emotional abuse in personal relationships. Through case studies and real-life examples, readers were encouraged to trust their instincts and seek support when faced with emotional abuse.

In Chapter 4, we explored the five cycles of emotional abuse. This chapter highlighted the repetitive nature of abusive relationships, emphasizing the importance of breaking the cycle. By understanding the patterns that perpetuate emotional abuse, readers gained valuable insights into the dynamics at play and were encouraged to seek help and break free from the cycle.

Chapter 5 addressed the six phases of healing from emotional abuse. Recognizing that healing is a process, this chapter provided a roadmap for individuals on their journey towards recovery. By acknowledging the pain, seeking support, and implementing self-care strategies, readers were empowered to reclaim their lives and move towards a healthier, happier future.

Finally, Chapter 6 discussed the crucial topic of knowing

when to walk away. Recognizing the complexity of leaving an emotionally abusive relationship, this chapter offered guidance and support to those contemplating making this difficult decision. By exploring various factors such as safety, self-worth, and personal boundaries, readers gained insight into the importance of prioritizing their well-being and taking steps towards a life free from abuse.

In conclusion, this book has endeavored to shed light on the insidious nature of emotional abuse, while providing practical tools and resources for those impacted by it. By understanding emotional abuse, identifying its signs, breaking the cycle, and embarking on a healing journey, readers are equipped with the knowledge and strength to reclaim their lives and cultivate healthy relationships. May this book serve as a guiding light for those seeking healing, empowerment, and a brighter future beyond the shadows of emotional abuse.

References

[1] Karakurt, G., & Silver, K. E. (2013). Emotional abuse in intimate relationships: The role of gender and age. Violence and victims, 28(5), 804-821. doi: 10.1891/0886-6708.vv-d-12-00041

[2] Rakovec-Felser, Z. (2014). Domestic violence and abuse in intimate relationship from public health perspective. Health psychology research, 2(3), 1821. doi: 10.4081/hpr.2014.1821

[3] Wagers, S. M. (2015). Deconstructing the "power and control motive": Moving beyond a unidimensional view of power in domestic violence theory. Partner Abuse, 6 (2), 230–242. DOI:10.1891/1946-6560.6.2.230

[4] Bond, S. B., & Bond, M. (2004). Attachment styles and violence within couples. The Journal of nervous and mental disease, 192(12), 857-863. DOI:10.1097/01.nmd.0000146879.33957.ec

[5] Psychcentral. (2022). Emotional Abuse Test. Retrieved from: https://psychcentral.com/quizzes/domestic-violence-quiz

[6] Chavis, A. Z., & Hill, M. S. (2008). Integrating multiple intersecting identities: A multicultural conceptualization of

the power and control wheel. Women & Therapy, 32(1), 121-149. DOI:10.1080/02703140802384552

[7] Safe Lives. (2020). Psychological Violence. Retrieved from:

https://www.safelivesresearch.org.uk/Comms/Psychologi cal%20Violence%20-%20Full%20Report.pdf

[8] Smullens, S. (2010). The codification and treatment of emotional abuse in structured group therapy. International journal of group psychotherapy, 60(1), 111-130.   DOI: 10.1521/ijgp.2010.60.1.111

[9] Thomas, S. (2016). Healing from Hidden Abuse: A Journey Through the Stages of Recovery from Psychological Abuse (Vol. 1). MAST Publishing House.

[10] Tyrrell, P., Harberger, S., Schoo, C., & Siddiqui, W. (2022). Kubler-Ross Stages of Dying and Subsequent Models of Grief. In StatPearls [Internet]. StatPearls Publishing.

Disclaimer

The information contained in this book and its components provide information and insights that the author has extensively researched and also experienced in practice. The author's postulations are personal recommendations, and reading this book does not guarantee identical results.

The author has taken reasonable measures to provide accurate and up-to-date information. However, neither the author nor their associates can be held responsible for any unintended errors or omissions.

It is important to note that this book may include third-party materials, which consist of opinions expressed by their respective owners. Therefore, the author does not assume liability for any third-party content or opinions.

The publication of third-party materials does not imply the author's endorsement of the information, products, services, or opinions contained therein. Using such materials does not guarantee matching results. The inclusion of third-party content is solely a recommendation and represents the author's personal opinion.

Due to the dynamic nature of the Internet and potential

changes in company policies and editorial guidelines, the accuracy and relevance of the information provided may evolve over time.

This book is copyrighted by Inspira, and all rights are reserved. Reproduction, copying, or creation of derivative works, whether in whole or in part, is strictly prohibited without the author's written permission.

www.ingramcontent.com/pod-product-compliance
Lightning Source LLC
Chambersburg PA
CBHW051833250726
48659CB00005B/1812